Strive to Overcome

DAN and LAURIE'S STORY

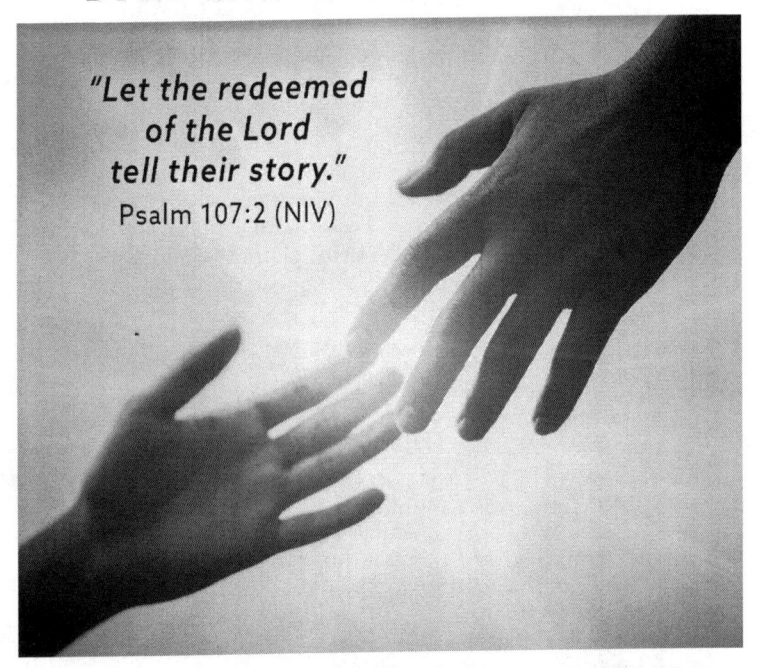

"Let the redeemed of the Lord tell their story."
Psalm 107:2 (NIV)

DAN and LAURIE OLSEN

Address all personal correspondence to:
Dan and Laurie Olsen
dannlaurie331@gmail.com

Individuals and church groups may order books from Dan and Laurie Olsen directly, or from the publisher. Retailers and wholesalers should order from our distributors. Refer to the Deeper Revelation Books website for distribution information, as well as an online catalog of all our books.

Published by:
Deeper Revelation Books
Revealing "the deep things of God" (1 Cor. 2:10)
P.O. Box 4260
Cleveland, TN 37320 423-478-2843
Website: www.deeperrevelationbooks.org
Email: info@deeperrevelationbooks.org

Deeper Revelation Books assist Christian authors in publishing and distributing their books. Final responsibility for design, content, permissions, editorial accuracy, and doctrinal views, either expressed or implied, belongs to the author. What you hold in your hands (or what you are viewing in an e-book format) is an expression of this author's passion to publish the truth with a spirit of excellence. It was a blessing and an honor to help in the process.

Table of Contents

PART 1

DAN'S TESTIMONY

CHAPTER 1

My Early Years

*G*od brought me into this world on August 30, 1956, the third child of my earthly parents, John and Ann Olsen. I am one of those somewhat rare people you meet in Prescott, Arizona, who was actually born and raised there. In fact, my grandma Elvizia, also known as "Grammy," my mom, and my son, Jeff, were also born there. Nearly every day, I give thanks to God for John and Ann Olsen, because even though it took me many years to fully accept Jesus Christ into my heart as my Lord and Savior, which I'll talk about later, God used them to build my foundation of faith.

They had me baptized as an infant and educated me at Sacred Heart Catholic School and Prescott High School. They provided a faith-based upbringing that was solid and loving in every way. They also instilled in me good manners, morals, and values. I was taught about the Creator, God the Father. They taught me Jesus Christ, His Son, came to this earth, was crucified, died, was buried, and ascended into heaven. They also taught me there was a Spirit, a part of God called the Holy Spirit, and taught me about sin and repentance. I attended church on a regular basis.

My childhood was great. Along with my sisters, Kathy and Marie, and my brother, Mike, I was raised in a loving home in which, from my perspective, God provided many blessings and few hardships. My family spent the school-year months in our Prescott home, the home my parents lived in until they passed, just below the intersection of White Spar and Copper Basin roads in Prescott. My cousins lived next door and my Grammy, great aunts, and great uncles lived in the "Big House" a stone's throw away.

They owned a grocery store, the Hassayampa Market, and "Grammy" was affectionately known to give all of us kids free ice cream or candy on a daily basis. Our summer months were spent on my dad's farm and ranch, the JCJ Ranch, located fifteen miles northwest of Paulden, Arizona. The things I learned at "The Ranch" have proved to be lifelong, invaluable lessons. What could be better for a kid, right?

One enormous thing was lacking, however. Even with all God's blessings of a great family and a wonderful childhood, through nobody's fault but my own, I had not accepted Jesus Christ into my heart, and I did not have a personal relationship with Him.

Strive To Overcome

CHAPTER 2

Boy to Man

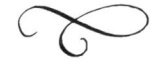

*A*fter high school, I made the decision to leave home and move out of state to attend college at Colorado State University. I looked at this transition as the time in my life I would grow from boy to man, and in some ways I did. However, the challenges of leaving the security of my parents (although they supported me financially) and facing the temptations of this fallen world alone led to times I am not very proud of. I quit going to church, partied and drank excessively, and almost flunked out my freshman year. By the grace of God and the values I had been taught (mainly to honor your father and mother, who were paying lots of money for my education), I buckled down and got my degree in Industrial Construction Management.

I took a job out of college in Houston, Texas, working on a skyscraper project in the downtown. I was doing well and rising in positions. However, my commitment to

God and my faith was pretty much nonexistent. So, like He often does because He knows best, God stepped in. It's a long and complicated story I won't go into, but I was fired!

Devastated and feeling like a complete failure, instead of turning to God, I called home and looked for my parents to feel sorry for me. But because He is such an awesome God, He gave me a clear and concise answer to what He wanted me to do. Of course, as parents my mom and dad were consoling me and feeling sorry for me, so God put my brother-in-law Steve, whom I barely knew at the time, on the phone. Steve told me to come home because he had a job for me. He and my sister needed a house built, and they wanted me to build it. WOW! I couldn't get home fast enough. God was definitely at work, but I didn't realize how this would change my life.

CHAPTER 3

God Gives Me a Career, My First Wife, and My Children

I came back to Prescott, moved back in with my parents, and spent the next eighteen months building two houses, one for my sister and the other for my brother. However, God had much more in His plan for my life. Not only did He bring me back to Prescott to build those houses, but He also gave me the opportunity to become part of Olsen's Grain, the family business.

Even with these blessings He was handing me, He had one of His most awesome blessings for me already involved in Olsen's Grain. Barb happened to be the first person that my brother and sister-in-law hired to help them in their Chino Valley store. This, my friends, was no coincidence. Barb and I became friends, and we leaned on each other. God then brought our hearts together, and we fell in love.

On September 28, 1985, God married us as one in the flesh at American Lutheran

Church. After our wedding, Barb and I became a part of the American Lutheran family, where we attended regularly until 2018.

God continued to bless us and strengthen our love for each other for thirty-three years. With my marriage to Barb came God's blessing of two wonderful stepdaughters, Kristi and Scoob, who accepted me as their dad in every way, shape, and form. In their eyes, I am their dad, and in my eyes, they are my kids. I love them both with all of my heart! Without a doubt, this is the way God wants it.

Through Kristi, God has also gifted me with an awesome son-in-law, Warren, and a wonderful granddaughter, Ally. But wait—God had still another great gift. On April 28, 1987, God blessed Barb and I with a child of our own. Jeff came to us in a miraculous way because Barb was forty-four when she gave birth to him. The world around us had doubts a woman her age could have a normal, healthy baby. But as we all know, "With God, all things are possible" (Matthew 19:26). This child came into the world strong, healthy, and smart. What a gift! God was definitely at work.

God continued to help us grow for the

next eighteen years as we finished raising Scoob, raised Jeff, and did our part to grow the family business. God's gift of Olsen's Grain and working with my siblings, whom I partner with, has always been a huge blessing in my life. It has allowed me to always be involved in our children's lives.

I thank God for my parents, wife, kids, grandchild, and siblings. He has blessed me in so many ways throughout my years. I am now able to realize how huge God's blessings have been, but that was not always the case. You see, through nobody's fault but my own, I still had not accepted Jesus Christ into my heart, and I did not have a personal relationship with Him. That all began to change when the first of God's three "wake up" calls rocked my world on April 1, 2005. Yes, April Fool's Day.

CHAPTER 4

My Miraculous Healing

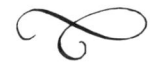

April 1st was a Friday, and we had made plans to meet another couple for dinner at a restaurant called The Office in downtown Prescott. I had never met this couple, but Barb had gotten to know Joneen, the wife, while doing volunteer work at Abia Judd School. I had not felt "right" for a couple of days but decided to go ahead with our plans.

At the restaurant, I sat down with excitement to meet new friends and enjoy a meal with them. We all ordered drinks and settled in for a time to get to know each other and enjoy each other's company. God, though, had a different plan! When my beer came, I took one sip and immediately knew that it was not staying down. I sprinted to the bathroom, feeling sicker than I had ever been.

When I was able to return to the table, I asked Barb to take me home. I was really sick. We excused ourselves, having made a good first impression on Rob and Joneen,

I'm sure, and headed home. As we passed the hospital, Barb asked if she should stop, and I said no. Well, I should have said yes because we were at the ER within a couple hours. My temperature was over 104 degrees, and I was really sick. The doctors got my fever down, did some tests, and sent me home. Over the next four days I visited the doctor a couple times where he tried some different things, but I didn't get any better.

On Wednesday I asked Barb to take me back to the ER, as something was really wrong. After testing me for everything under the sun, at about 5:00 p.m. the doctors finally concluded I had acute hepatitis A and would have to be admitted.

The last thing I remember from the next several days is a vague recollection of my family coming to see me late Wednesday evening. The rest of the story comes from what Barb and my kids have told me.

On Thursday a doctor, I'm not sure which one, removed my IV, thinking I was getting better. Barb questioned this and summoned my dad. My dad called for a specialist, Dr. Milt, who immediately ordered the IV put back in.

When Barb came into my room on Friday

morning, she told me I couldn't speak very well and couldn't stand or walk. She called Dr. Milt's office. The staff told her Dr. Milt was off that day, but they would call him. Soon thereafter, Dr. Milt's partner came in and reported that Dr. Milt had determined toxins from my liver were affecting my brain. I needed to be flown to Phoenix for a liver transplant, and I may end up with brain damage.

I can't even begin to imagine how Barb must have felt about this news. What she tells me is God gave her the strength and courage to make two calls. The first call was to Prescott High School to summon Jeff out of class to drive her to Phoenix. Jeff, only seventeen at the time, stepped up for God and completely took over my role in helping his mother. No doubt God was using Jeff, and even though I am sure it was very hard for him, I am confident this trial was God's instrument to grow him and make him strong.

The second call was to my brother to come to Yavapai Regional Medical Center to support my elderly parents who were to stay with me until the helicopter left with me in it. Later Barb told me, "I don't know how Mike got from Chino Valley to Prescott so fast, but he was there in no time." Again, it was another case of a family member stepping up for God in this trying ordeal.

When I arrived at Good Samaritan Hospital by helicopter several hours later (it seems the hospital didn't have a bed available right away), the news got worse. Barb, Jeff, Scoob, Kristi, and my baby granddaughter Ally were waiting as the helicopter brought me to the roof. They did not know if I was dead or alive, but after seeing me rushed down the hall in a frantic manner, it was evident I was still hanging on.

I have absolutely no recollection of this helicopter ride, but the flight nurse later told Scoob I was trying to kick the door open. Evidently, I was very combative and acting like a crazy madman.

After a couple hours of working on me, I was brought to the ICU where the medical staff strapped me to my bed. Soon thereafter, someone on the medical staff approached Barb, Scoob, and Jeff and informed them it didn't look like I was going to make it through the night. If I did, I would definitely have to have a liver transplant, and my brain might fall into a coma.

But God had a different plan! First of all, He gave Barb the strength to look that person in the eye and state, "That is not an option!" I had a breathing tube and seven IVs pumping meds into me, but I was still alive and did make it through the night.

On Saturday morning, Scoob was in the room with me as I lay lifeless except for my chest going up and down from the breathing machine. She told me I looked like a breathing corpse.

That's when God intervened. By this time word of my sickness had spread throughout Prescott, and many, many people were praying for me. Pastor Eunice entered my hospital room, laid her hands on me, and began to pray. Scoob told me my body flinched, and from that moment on I started getting better. My vital signs began to improve, and the liver transplant was put on hold.

I slowly but steadily improved over the next couple days, and on Tuesday morning I woke up to the smiling face of my bride. However, it took me a few minutes to focus and realize who she was and where I was. My mom and brother arrived shortly thereafter. I recall being able get out of bed and sit in a chair.

Later in the afternoon I was moved out of the ICU and onto a different floor. The next day my daughter Kristi and her husband Warren came just to visit me, or so they thought. God had a different plan. By that afternoon, only four days after the doctors were ready to write me off, they released me. You see, God had sent Kristi and Warren, not to visit, but to take Barb and me home. God had healed me, no doubt in my mind! Praise Him!

CHAPTER 5

Jesus Guides Me Through Recovery

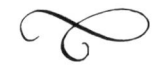

*J*ohn 3:5–8 says "Very truly I tell you, no one can enter the kingdom of God unless they are born of water and the Spirit. Flesh gives birth to flesh, but the Spirit gives birth to spirit. You should not be surprised at my saying, 'You must be born again.' The wind blows wherever it pleases. You hear its sound, but you cannot tell where it comes from or where it is going. So it is with everyone born of the Spirit."

I was healed but still had to recover and figure out what God had just done for me. I was very weak. I had lost about forty pounds and was yellow from jaundice. As I began to recover, the Holy Spirit went to work on me. The first thing He did was use Barb to explain to me that I was still physically alive by His grace. I had been on my way out, but He slammed the door shut. He wanted me to remain in this world for a purpose, and I needed to find out what that reason was.

After a few days of still feeling pretty sick, I began to take small walks to build my strength. As I walked, I talked to God. Each day the walks and the talks got longer until they increased to an hour and a half. I got stronger and better every day, and the Holy Spirit began to push me toward a personal relationship with Jesus Christ. I was to be born again of His Spirit. I began to seek Him through reading the Bible daily, connecting with Him in educational classes and books, and enjoying His presence in my life with other Christians in small groups.

It was during this time I truly began to believe in Jesus Christ and receive His free gift of salvation into everlasting life. I invited Him into my heart, repenting of all the sins in my past and finally turning from my sinful behavior. By the grace of God and as He promised, I had been born again, recreated in the image of my Savior.

You see, it wasn't that I didn't believe in Jesus. I did, but I had not invited Him into my heart and chosen to receive the gift He offers to all, the free gift of salvation and eternal life, which begins the minute we take this step.

Wow! When I finally made this decision

that no one else could do for me, my life changed. I now knew without a shadow of doubt that even though I could expect many more trials and tribulations in my life, I could face them with the power of the Holy Spirit and with a peace in my heart that goes beyond all understanding.

John 3:16–18 says, "For God so loved the world that he gave his one and only Son, that whoever believes in him shall not perish but have eternal life. For God did not send his Son into the world to condemn the world, but to save the world through him. Whoever believes in him is not condemned, but whoever does not believe stands condemned already because they have not believed in the name of God's one and only Son."

I began to walk with Jesus daily as He guided me down the path of preparation for what He had planned for me. I was back at work at Olsen's Grain, but it was very clear to me He had put people in place to take over my day-to-day role in the company. You see, God had a different plan, but I was resisting going all in for His purposes.

I was not getting the picture of what He wanted me to do, so He gave me another nudge with a second wake-up call. One of our family traditions is to travel to Glamis, California, and ride our quads on the Imperial Sand Dunes. We set out on one of these ventures on March 11, 2007. Barb, Jeff, and I traveled from Prescott, and Warren, Kristi, and Ally from Flagstaff.

As we approached Peeples Valley, my phone rang. The phone indicated it was Warren, but when Barb answered, a complete stranger was on the line. This person told Barb there had been a terrible accident, and she had called to inform us that our kids' truck had crashed.

At this point, Warren got on the phone and told us he was all right and it appeared that Ally and Kristi would be okay too. However, the ambulance was coming to take them all to the hospital back in Flagstaff.

We turned our rig around and beelined it back home where we changed vehicles and headed for Flagstaff. We were all praying God had protected them, but we also knew we might find tragic circumstances when we got to the hospital. What we found when we got there was that our awesome God had protected them, and the worst of the injuries was a badly broken wrist for Kristi. In fact, we found little three-year-old

Ally racing up and down the hallway with her bare little bottom showing out the back of her hospital gown.

When we talked to Kristi, she revealed to us how God was truly in the picture protecting them. She told us about an angel God had sent to her the night before. It was late, dark, and cold as Kristi was closing the Olsen's Grain store she and Warren manage. As she approached the door to lock it, a lady appeared. This lady apologized for keeping Kristi late but said she needed feed for her animals. She then asked if she could wash her hands because she had been working all day teaching people how to properly install a car seat. Kristi asked her, "What's the big deal? You put the car seat in place and buckle it in."

"Oh no," the lady replied. "There is more to it than that. You must climb in, put your full weight in the seat, and cinch it as tightly as you can."

Kristi replied, "I didn't know that, but I will be sure and do it that way from now on."

The next morning as they prepared to leave on their trip, Kristi climbed in, put her full weight in the seat, and cinched it up a good three more inches. At this point Ally asked her mom why she was in her car seat.

Well, no one knew it at the time, but this no doubt saved Ally's life. When the dust settled after the wreck that happened within the next hour, the cab of the truck rested a mere one inch from Ally's head. There was no doubt in my mind God had given my family another miracle!

CHAPTER 6

God Uses My Two Guardian Angels Again

*G*od continued to strengthen me and bring me closer to Him through my personal relationship with Jesus. I was walking daily with Jesus, growing in His Word, exercising every morning, and feeling better than ever.

Then in April 2009, four years after my bout with hepatitis A, my doctor prescribed a colonoscopy. The nurses prepped me for the procedure and connected me to the heart monitor. As the medical team was getting me ready, the nurse in charge looked into my eyes and asked me what was going on with my heart. Dumbfounded, I replied nothing was going on that I knew of. As far as I knew, my heart has always been strong.

"No," she replied, "something is definitely not right. We'll have to see what Dr. Milt has to say when he comes in."

Yes, this was the same Dr. Milt who had sent me to Phoenix to see the liver specialist when the toxins were going into my brain. God had put him once again in a position to save my life. He said, "We'll go ahead with this procedure because we are monitoring your heart, but you must get to your doctor ASAP." He then completed the colonoscopy and sent me home.

However, early the next morning Dr. Milt called and told me he was very worried about me. He couldn't sleep and had already arranged an appointment for me with a cardiologist that day.

The cardiologist quickly determined my heart had developed an irregular rhythm called ventricular tachycardia. That rhythm can be fatal if the heart stays in it too long. He told me, "You can thank Dr. Milt for saving your life because you are a walking time bomb."

He had a solution, however. He could implant a pacemaker-defibrillator that would correct the rhythm and keep me safe if the heart had to be shocked back into a normal rhythm. So on April 28, 2009, my son's twenty-second birthday, my new lifelong companion was implanted into my chest.

Again, God had used Dr. Milt to keep me on this earth.

Aside from doing physical work too soon and needing to be shocked—and I mean the-world-is-coming-to-an-end shocked—I have been healthy ever since. God definitely had my attention now, but He still had to directly speak to me through someone else.

Enter again, Pastor Eunice! She had come back into my life after me not seeing her for a couple years as she was leading a church in another state. She had returned to Prescott, and Barb and I were helping her start a new church.

One day out of the blue, Pastor Eunice said to me, "Dan, the Lord told me He wants you to be a leader for Him in men's ministry. He has big plans for you in leading men. Check out Every Man Ministries on the internet."

It was then the Holy Spirit took over. He set me on fire to be a servant leader for Him in this ministry. Within a few weeks I was in California being trained at Every Man Ministries on how to connect men to God and to each other.

The Holy Spirit inspired me to come up with a plan. I spent the entire drive back from

California talking and listening to God. He laid it on my heart to invite men to a weekly gathering, including fellowship, Bible study, and breakfast.

I met with Pastor Eunice and explained what God was leading me to do. She was elated, but she encouraged me to bring it to the leadership of American Lutheran Church because the plan was much better suited to become a ministry there rather than at her church.

The lead pastor and church council at American Lutheran Church loved the idea, and Crossfire Men's Ministry was launched, developing into a ministry that continues to connect men to God and to each other. The Holy Spirit also led me to raise up men in my circle of influence to capture the vision of what He wanted in the Prescott area. Through God's grace and to His honor, several men's conferences and events have been held, and many men have been connected to God and to other men.

CHAPTER 7

God's Calling and Protection

I attended a Young Life men's camp and had the pleasure of being led through the weekend study sessions by a very inspirational speaker named Bill Paige. The few men I attended with were some of my closest brothers in Christ. We all collectively decided we must bring Bill Paige to Prescott to speak to the men in our area so they, too, could be inspired in their walk with Christ, just as we were. The Lord inspired me to take the lead in what I thought would simply be inviting Bill Paige to come to a church where we would gather as many as possible to hear him speak.

But again, God had a different plan. I inquired to see if this was something Mr. Paige would be interested in doing. He agreed to it and gave me his price. I then gathered the men who had attended the camp with me for lunch to discuss whether to move forward or not with this idea. Well, the Holy

Spirit moved powerfully and quickly in these men, and by the time lunch was over, we were planning a men's expo. I was to lead it. Not only would it include Bill Paige as the keynote speaker but also a free breakfast and lunch, interactive games that appeal to men, vendor booths with "guy things," and worship music.

We began meeting together to pray, plan, raise funds, and form a nonprofit corporation to conduct our business under. It was a huge undertaking, but we were empowered by the Holy Spirit. The first expo was scheduled for September 8, 2012. We named it the "Get Real Men's Expo" because Bill Paige's underlying message to us men was to "get real" with Jesus.

September 8th that year was the first Saturday after Labor Day weekend. As God's chosen leader of the Get Real Men's Expo, I had worked tirelessly preparing for it and was ready for a relaxing time with my family over the long weekend. We all decided to spend the weekend in the mountains at Happy Jack, Arizona.

Well, the trip turned out to be anything but relaxing. Once again, we had a horrific accident, and once again, God stepped in and protected my granddaughter and me! We decided to take a day trip from Happy Jack to Blue Mesa Reservoir. It was a short drive, and Ally wanted me to drive her in our side-by-side. So we set out, Ally and I ahead in the side-by-side and Kristi, Warren, Scoob, and Barb in the pickup truck following us. Ally and I had gotten ahead of them as they stopped to visit with a friend along the road who was the sheriff on patrol that day.

As we tooled along, I thought I saw a wild turkey off to the side, so I turned my head to look back. When I did this, I slowly veered off the road, and we rolled multiple times approximately seventy-five feet into the canyon. This is where God intervened. A huge, downed pine tree stopped the multiple rollovers, and we came to rest upside down.

I felt no injury, and Ally said she was okay too. The helmets and roll cage had done what they are designed to do, but if the dead tree had not been there, we would have dropped another 100 feet over a dry waterfall into a bed of rocks! I have no doubt in my mind God put that tree there. He also showed our family members where we had crashed, or they would have gone to the reservoir and not been able to find us. They would not have had any idea where to look.

Immediately after the dust from the wreck settled, I could hear the pickup rattling down the rough road. I instructed Ally to scream as loudly as she could, and I started whistling. By God's grace, Warren heard what he knew was his daughter's scream, and Barb caught a glimpse of the red machine down in the canyon. Warren and Scoob were on us in the blink of an eye and helped us climb out to the road. There was no cell service, but Kristi hustled back to the sheriff friend, and the EMS arrived quickly.

They hauled us into a hospital in Flagstaff, but neither of us had any injuries at all. We were released and sent on our way. Praise the Lord!

The enemy definitely wanted to take the leader of the Get Real Men's Expo out in an attempt to stop 800 men from gathering in the name of Jesus, but God said NO, that isn't going to happen. Under God's using me in its leadership role, the Get Real Men's Expo continued to be a premier Christian event for men in the Prescott area for ten years. God also continued to have me lead Crossfire Men's Ministry for nine years. All praise and glory to Him!

CHAPTER 8

My Years of Tribulation

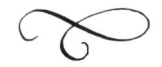

*A*lthough the years leading up to 2012 had their times of trials and tribulations, they also had many, many, many blessings. The biggest blessing was me being recreated in God's image when I surrendered it all to my Lord and Savior Jesus Christ in 2005. Because those earlier years were so blessed, I look at the years between 2012 and 2018 as my most turbulent ones. Not because of health issues, even though I was diagnosed with bladder cancer. The cancer didn't even concern me because I now knew God was in control of life, and I had a peace about it. I just knew God would heal me if it was His will. It was His will; I've never had an issue with this cancer and didn't have to endure chemo or radiation. Doctors just cut the cancerous part out, and that was it!

However, what did happen during these years tested my faith and trust in God to the core. You see, Satan got a stranglehold on Barb through his evil vice of alcohol. She slowly slipped into addiction before I recognized it. But once I did, I tried everything the world tells you to do with an addicted loved one. I prayed, but I did not totally surrender her to God and His will. Alcohol addiction completely changed Barb. I agonized for years as I dealt with this person I didn't even know anymore but yet was married to.

For those of you who have never had to deal with an addicted loved one, I can't even begin to explain how extremely difficult and heartbreaking it can be. I had to endure lots of verbal abuse as well as many hours of watching my wife try to live life in a drunken stupor. It was very hard. However, years before, I had vowed to take care of her in sickness and in health. I knew caring for her is what God wanted me to do, even though in my flesh I wanted to give up many times.

But God would not let me give up. He put people in my life to help me persevere. He used my kids and wonderful brothers and sisters in Christ to hold me accountable to God's Word. The emotional support of these people got me through the very tough years of loving and taking care of Barb. I could not have done it without all of them.

Eventually in 2017, after getting help and

staying sober for two years, Barb relapsed and started drinking again during our move to a new house. She soon started losing her cognitive skills and was diagnosed with dementia. Within a couple months she was no longer safe to drive, or even to be alone, so the Lord sent me an angel in the form of a caregiver for Barb. This wonderful person befriended Barb and spent months taking her on rides and just being her friend.

She was a godsend because during this time God called me in to a completely different ministry as a hospice chaplain. Several years earlier at a men's ministry conference, I had answered God's call to become a chaplain, not knowing how or when He would use this in my life. Now I knew. Working with end-of-life patients was therapy for me and prepared me to handle Barb's eventual death with grace and total trust in God. Yes, I had been involved in hospital chaplaincy, and I had walked through the deaths of both my parents, but I knew God had something very special for me through hospice chaplaincy.

The caregiver took care of Barb during the day, and I took care of her at night. The dementia would not let her eat, as her brain told her she was stuffed after one or two bites. Barring life support, which Barb had long ago rejected when she was totally coherent, and barring a miracle of God, Barb's body was going to wither away and die.

That is exactly what happened. She eventually became too weak to function, ended up bedridden, and passed away at a mere seventy pounds on January 24, 2019. The good news was she had long ago accepted Jesus Christ as her Lord and Savior and asked for forgiveness of her sins. She is now dancing on the streets of gold in heaven. I believe with all my heart that Satan used his evil vice of alcohol addiction to steal Barb's mind and body, but he did not steal her soul because Jesus had already purchased her soul on the cross. Now she lives with Him for eternity!

CHAPTER 9

God's Most Special Gift to Me

*I*n the fall of 2018, two significant events happened that set my life on a new course. However, the first would not come to a full understanding and fruition until after Barb's passing. The first thing that happened started with a request from a fellow brother in Christ, my fellow chaplain and co-worker at Kindred Hospice. He approached me and said he had a patient named Jon Lindquist out in Chino Valley he could not connect with. God had a different plan in mind. He then asked me to take Jon on as a patient to see if Jon would respond to me.

So on my birthday, August 30, 2018, I made a trip out to Chino Valley and met with Jon and his wife, Laurie. Laurie was a Christian, but Jon was not. Through God's grace, I connected well with both Jon and Laurie. Through the power of the Holy Spirit, God used Laurie and I to bring Jon to an understanding of Jesus Christ and what He did for all of us to save us from eternal damnation. About a week before Jon lost consciousness from a six-year battle with colon cancer, he accepted Jesus as his Lord and Savior and repented of his sins. Jon lives! Praise Jesus!

A couple weeks after Jon's passing, Laurie held a small celebration of life for Jon which she asked me to officiate. It was an honor for me. Laurie and I parted ways believing we may never cross paths again. Guess what? God had a different plan!

It was soon after this, in November 2018, God shook up my world again. I was continuing to serve as a hospice chaplain, take care of Barb, and lead the men's ministry at American Lutheran Church. However, this time the Holy Spirit convicted me of a sin in my heart I did not want to own up to. You see, a good friend, who was a married woman, and I had allowed our friendship to grow into something that went beyond what was appropriate for two people who were married. It was an emotional affair in which I was coveting the love of another man's wife. That was my sin.

However, in His grace, after repenting and turning from my sin by completely severing all ties with this friend, God forgave me. He then moved me out of American Lutheran, which had been my church home for thirty-three years. He called me to Mountaintop Christian Fellowship where another friend and confidant was the pastor. God wanted me to serve Him in men's ministry at this church. It was a big change many of my friends at American Lutheran did not understand, but it was definitely God's will and where God wanted me. It was also where God wanted Barb's celebration of life held. God made that clear to me for reasons I didn't understand at the time, but I prayed, and by the power of the Holy Spirit, I obeyed His direction. I can now look back and clearly see how God was going to bless me.

Soon after Barb passed, I got a text from Laurie Lindquist expressing her condolences. When I received that text, the Holy Spirit inspired me to call Laurie. I knew I had failed to do any follow up with Laurie after Jon's passing. Her text reminded me of her, and I reached out. I thanked her for her heartfelt message and invited her to Barb's service. She asked where it was going to be held. I told her it would be at Mountaintop, a non-denominational, Bible-teaching church, and God inspired her to attend.

Laurie had spent the four months since Jon's passing looking for a church but never connected with one. However, when she walked into Mountaintop, God clearly spoke to her and said this was the church He wanted her in. Laurie loved Mountaintop's style of worship and the preaching of my pastor friend. However, she never dreamed God wanted her at Mountaintop to reconnect with me because He wanted to gift us with each other! This was not in Laurie's plan. In fact, she had vowed to her family and friends that after experiencing the physical death of two husbands, she was never getting married again. But God had a different plan!

On Sunday, February 10, 2019, Laurie came back to Mountaintop to praise and worship her Lord. When I walked in, I saw her sitting alone near the back of the church. Figuring she didn't know anyone else, I went over to her and asked if she'd mind if I sat with her. She greeted me with a warm smile and told me I could. I made sure I left a seat between us so no one would think I already had a girlfriend so soon after my wife's passing.

As we were singing and worshiping, I noticed tears rolling down Laurie's cheeks and was concerned she was still struggling with Jon's passing. The Holy Spirit inspired me to ask Laurie to lunch after church to catch up and talk about life as recently widowed individuals. She accepted my invitation. Praise the Lord!

When we sat down for lunch, I learned those tears were tears of joy because God was moving in her life. Oh wow, she had no idea how He was going to move in both our lives. During our conversation, God clearly showed us how equally yoked we were spiritually. He showed us how like-minded we were and how many interests we had in common.

We spent a couple hours visiting, and when it was time to part, we hugged each other, and both of us left wondering what God was doing. Now we see this lunch date was clearly the beginning of God's plan for Dan Olsen and Laurie Lindquist! We got together again two days later when Laurie reached out to me to help her with a vehicle problem. After taking care of the problem, we visited for another couple of hours. This time when we parted, we kissed passionately, and our hearts melted for each other.

Two days after that, Valentine's Day, I asked Laurie to be my valentine and meet me for lunch. We both had not dated for many years, and Laurie didn't know what to think when I sat across the table from her. She had bought me a Valentine's Day card and a small gift. We had an enjoyable time as we engaged in a great conversation about living life as followers of Jesus Christ. Laurie and I both knew we were a match put together by the Lord Himself and our new-found relationship would continue.

However, I left on a ski trip with Jeff the next day and Laurie on a trip to her place on the Colorado River near Blythe, California. Even though we were apart, both of us had the other on our minds, and we texted and spoke on the phone many times over the next few days.

When I headed home, Laurie invited me to stop by and said she would have dinner waiting for me. Of course, I accepted and couldn't wait to see her again. Laurie and I started going to church together and spent every evening together over the next two months. We fell deeply in love, and, taking nothing away from Barb or Jon, this love was incredibly different. This love was put together by God Almighty!

We knew without a doubt we were to spend our final season of life together, married by Him, one in the flesh. We knew we were to honor God and get married quickly without living together. We were to do this His way, and we were convicted to obey Him! We were married, one in the flesh, by God on March 31, 2019.

Acts 5:29-32 says, "Peter and the other apostles replied: 'We must obey God rather than human beings! The God of our ancestors raised Jesus from the dead—whom you killed by hanging him on a cross. God exalted him to his own right hand as Prince and Savior that he might bring Israel to repentance and forgive their sins. We are witnesses of these things, and so is the Holy Spirit, whom God has given to those who obey him.'"

PART 2

LAURIE'S TESTIMONY

CHAPTER 10
From Little Girl to a Business-Owning, Married Mom

*I*was born in Escondido, California, in 1958, to George and Betty Burkhardt. I was my father's only biological child, but my half-brother Bob and my half-sister Sue were, and still are, very special to me. Life was good as a little kid. I was definitely my daddy's little girl!

However, around the time I turned five, my parents started having problems and ended up divorcing. But my dad fought for me, and after a long, drawn-out ordeal, he won full custody of me. This was a miracle and definitely a gift from God because in 1963 a single dad getting custody of a little girl was unheard of.

My mother went on to marry her boy-friend. My relationship with her was very strained as her new husband didn't want me anywhere near them. He had a huge dislike for my father, which carried over onto me. Even at such a young age, God was taking care of me. As I look back, I can say without a doubt God had a plan for my life.

I was raised in San Diego. My father remarried, and with his new wife, Harriett, came two children, Bob and Carol, whom she and her ex-husband had adopted. Also, with my dad's marriage to Harriett, God brought her brother into my life, my beloved Uncle Don.

When I was seventeen, my father, stepmother, and her two children moved to Albuquerque, New Mexico, where my father and his lifelong friend went into partnership and bought a plating business. I did not want to move, so my dad graciously allowed me to stay in San Diego and live with my uncle and aunt. I lived with them for two years, and they were very good to me.

My Uncle Don became a second father to me, but the time did come for me to move to Albuquerque to be with my father. I thought my world had ended, but God knew what was best, and He was taking care of me. However, I must say, moving from Southern California to Albuquerque was quite the culture shock!

My move to Albuquerque took place

midway through my senior year in high school. As God's plan would have it, I settled into life in Albuquerque quickly, and God soon introduced me to the man that would not only lead me into a relationship with Jesus but also become my husband, Tom Cantrell. Tom and I fell in love and dated for a few months.

In June 1976, I graduated from high school and married Tom on July 10. God brought Tom into my life for many reasons, and as I've already mentioned, he ultimately led me to the Lord. I was not raised in church and had no knowledge of the many blessings our Lord has to offer His children as believers.

We had our trials but had a wonderful marriage. In October of 1980, we were blessed with our greatest gift, a daughter, Tammy. Tom and I vowed again that the only way out of this marriage was death.

At that time, Tom was the love of my life. I was drawn to Tom's love for the Lord and also wanted the light that shone in him. When Tammy was about three, we wanted her to know our heavenly Father. This world is a hard place, and we wanted her to know, no matter what, her heavenly Father loved her!! We searched for a church and started attending Tabernacle of Praise in Albuquerque. That is where I really came to know Jesus Christ and accept Him as my Savior. A whole new world opened up for me.

This is the church where Tammy went to school from kindergarten through the twelfth grade. As a newly born-again Christian, I had much to learn, so I began teaching Sunday school. I learned along with the children.

My father was having problems with his business partner, and I had been working in my father's business. To make a long story short, Tom and I purchased the business through the bankruptcy court. We only purchased the assets, and then applied for a small business loan and transformed the shop from automotive plating to industrial, mostly for aerospace parts. Building up the business took several years, but God blessed our hard work with a successful and thriving company.

CHAPTER 11

God Calls My Husband to His Eternal Home

om was blessed with a competitive love and skill for racing boats, so in 1983 he decided to start drag boat racing at a professional level in the class of Blown Alcohol Hydro. Our boat was Beautiful Noise. A racer's motto, no matter what he is racing, is that it is never fast enough!

Ultimately Tom stepped up into Top Fuel Hydro, which is the fastest class. The first couple years were tough, as we blew up a lot of parts (and money). However, in time, he climbed to the top of his class and was very competitive. He was a good example of a Christian racer.

When he decided to step up in class, I knew the risks and prayed about it a lot. In April 1997 in Phoenix, Tom set the world record, 241.96 miles per hour in a quarter mile on a single propeller. He had previously set several track records, but this was his first and only world record.

It was a huge step for our team, and owning a world record felt great, but that accomplishment did not diminish the dangers of the sport. I continued to ask our Lord to keep him safe. One Sunday in church as I was praying, I saw Tom crashing. Then I saw God put His hand out, and the boat was in God's hand. God gently put His hand in the water with the boat in it, all in one piece. I always took that to mean God would take care of him. Maybe Tom would suffer a few broken bones, but it would be nothing we couldn't deal with.

On July 10, 1997, Tom and I celebrated our twenty-first wedding anniversary. Two days later, on July 12, we were racing in Chowchilla, California. It was a Saturday evening when we buckled Tom in and set Beautiful Noise into the water for a qualifying pass. Tom looked Tammy and I in the eyes and said, "See you on the other side."

Those were Tom's last words to us because he had a horrific crash. Although "seeing us on the other side" hasn't come yet, we know without a doubt it will when we see him in heaven!

Tom was unconscious when the rescue team retrieved him from the water and brought him to the shore to assess his injuries. They would quickly determine he must be flown to the nearest trauma hospital in Fresno, California, and we would not be able to go with him. God intervened and provided a ride to Fresno for Tammy and I through our wonderful Christian friend and chaplain for Racers for Christ, Jim Jack. The Beautiful Noise crew stayed behind to gather and secure all the equipment and what was left of the race boat.

As Tammy and I arrived at the hospital, we were ushered in to meet with the doctors, who informed us Tom would need exploratory surgery to find out where he was bleeding internally and what, if anything, could be done to save his life. So as Tom went into surgery, the medical personnel ushered Tammy and I to the surgical waiting room.

On the way we passed the wife of another fellow racer in the hallway. She informed me her husband, who had crashed his boat in the same race about three hours prior to Tom's crash, had been pronounced dead. She was so angry with God, and I remember wondering how anyone could get through a tragedy like this without God. It was only the power of the Holy Spirit within me that gave me the courage to face the news to come.

The doctors came out of surgery and told us it was very bad and they had only seen internal injuries this severe in professional boxers. An investigation concluded the oxygen bottle in the boat that was there to protect Tom and keep him breathing in the event the boat sank had come loose from its mount and literally beat him up. The doctors also informed us they didn't think he would live through the beating his body had suffered.

After hearing this news, I remember going into prayer and reminding God about His promise to me through my vision in church that if Tom ever crashed, He would put His hand out, catch the boat, and gently set it back down onto the water. I said, "Do You remember, God?" I was sure God was going to save Tom for us.

However, God had a different plan, and I knew I had to let Tom go to his eternal home with his Savior, Jesus. By the power of the Holy Spirit, I told Tom it was okay to go be with the Lord. His body died on Monday, July 14, 1997, at about 1:00 p.m. when his ventilator tube kinked, and he went into cardiac arrest. At thirty-nine I became a widow! My husband, the love of my life and my daughter's daddy, was gone. Life as Tammy and I knew it turned completely upside down.

I had always taken comfort in what God had shown me in prayer and knew He would take care of Tom. I just couldn't understand how this could happen. I thought Tom would maybe sustain some injuries, but not death! However, God's plan is always perfect, and He did save Tom by bringing him to his eternal home in heaven. No, God didn't save my husband in the way I wanted Him to, but I do believe He saved Tom from something only He knew about. When Tom was young, he had polio, and I have often wondered if maybe it was coming back, which likely would have crippled him.

The next year was a huge adjustment for us. I often asked, "Dear Lord, how are Tammy and I supposed to survive?" When we left the hospital after Tom's passing to head to the funeral home to make arrangements, Tricia Yearwood's song "How Do I Live [Without You]?" came on the radio. Twenty-six years later, that song still speaks to me and touches my heart. I have no doubt God played that song for me at the precise moment I needed to hear it.

We returned home, and I sold our plating business, our silk-screening business, and all of our racing equipment. (Or I should say the equipment that didn't get destroyed in the accident.) I had spare motors and many spare parts, along with the semi and trailer set up for racing. Unfortunately, Tammy and I saw the worst in people during this time. Many thought we should sell them valuable equipment for next to nothing; some even thought I should give them Tom's stuff.

Several attorneys kept contacting me to file a blanket lawsuit against everyone involved in boat racing. But inspired by the Holy Spirit, I rejected their advice, knowing that Scripture is clear in Romans 12:19 where it says, "Do not take revenge, my dear friends, but leave room for God's wrath, for it is written: 'It is mine to avenge; I will repay,' says the Lord." Tom knew the risk every time he crawled into that race boat, and suing people over his accident would not bring him back. Tom and I had many discussions of the "what ifs," and we had agreed we wouldn't ever do anything to ruin the sport.

So I stood firm, obeyed, and tried to be a good steward of what God had blessed us with. I knew God would want me to keep my sixteen-year-old daughter in her private Christian school and change as little as possible in her life. I just tried to keep living, breathing, and putting one foot in front of the other. We had done everything together as a family. We worked together, lived together, and raced together. Tammy was a huge daddy's girl. When not at school or a school function, she was with us. She would spend a lot of time with her daddy at the shop learning the business or working on the race boat. We didn't know how to live without Tom, so Tammy went through a tough time trying to live without her daddy. Tom felt the sun rose and set with her. Tammy could do no wrong in her daddy's eyes. I can't express how hard all this was for Tammy and me to go through. Only with God's help did we have a chance, and God did provide me the strength I needed. But then I began to stumble and fall.

Strive To Overcome

CHAPTER 12
Walking the Broken Road

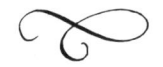

Over the next ten years, I was very angry with God. How could He take a good Christian man, a good husband, father, provider, and man who so loved the Lord? In my anger, I stumbled through some pretty stupid things. In that time Tammy met and married her husband. Dan was, and still is, very good to her. Thank God that He put Dan in her life at the right moment. God was there when I was falling. God took care of Tammy when He put Dan in her life. Her mother was in no shape to take care of anyone.

When Tammy left home, I did not lead a very Christian life, to put it mildly. I am not very proud of my actions as I walked the broken road, but I always loved the Lord. In June 2002 God blessed me with the second greatest gift of all, my granddaughter Lacie. She was, and still is, so much fun to be with. I never knew God could open my heart so much and fill it with so much love. I wanted to get right with God and be the grandmother God wanted me to be. When I held that precious baby for the first time and took a look at that gift from God, I felt so much love. That tiny little girl showed me she and her mother are my most special gifts from God. God was always there for me. He let me stumble but never left me.

By this time, I was living in Ruidoso, New Mexico, and went to work at a real estate company in their office. I worked with a woman named Alice, who was married to Charles, a pastor in a local church. I am very sure God put me there. Charles and Alice helped me see I wasn't leading the life God had planned for me.

I started going back to church and seeking the Lord. My life was still in disarray, so I had to clean house and seek the Lord's will for me. I had come to the truth that God did take care of Tom by taking him home. It just wasn't in the way I thought He should take care of him. That was a huge step for me in getting my relationship right with the Lord ... He did love me, and He had great things for me.

In John 14:15–21, Jesus says this:

"If you love me, keep my commands. And I will ask the Father, and he will

give you another advocate to help you and be with you forever—the Spirit of truth. The world cannot accept him, because it neither sees him nor knows him. But you know him, for he lives with you and will be in you. I will not leave you as orphans; I will come to you. Before long, the world will not see me anymore, but you will see me. Because I live, you also will live. On that day you will realize that I am in my Father, and you are in me, and I am in you. Whoever has my commands and keeps them is the one who loves me. The one who loves me will be loved by my Father, and I too will love them and show myself to them."

CHAPTER 13

God's Blessing, a Test, and Then Another Blessing

*G*od then put Jon Lindquist back in my life, and in 2010 I married him, never dreaming I would have to go through burying another husband. We had dated for about two years during the time I was attending high school and living in San Diego with my Uncle Don. God was working in my life again because I was seeking His will for me.

Jon and I were married for about eighteen months when we found out he had stage four colon cancer. God placed me in Jon's life for a reason. Jon had no children or anyone else to care for him. I sought the Lord's guidance and grace, and through me, God cared for Jon. However, Jon was tough and endured a lot. He went through several rounds of chemotherapy and radiation. Slowly these treatments destroyed some of his organs to the point they quit working and had to be removed.

At one point he had a colostomy. As he

was recovering, he developed a high fever, so I rushed him to the emergency room. He had gone septic. The doctors operated again and removed some of his colon. Jon was in the ICU on a ventilator, and I remember thinking, no God, not again! Tom's ventilator had kinked and sent him into cardiac arrest. Please don't let the same thing happen to Jon!

God didn't let that happen, and Jon made it through with hopes his colon could be reconnected at some point. However, it was not to be. He had another surgery where the doctors tried to reattach it, but he had too much damage, making a reconnection impossible. It was so hard for me to break this news to Jon, but God gave me the strength, and he accepted it.

As the years of treatment passed, God was always there by my side. Jon and I would remember the first years of our marriage when we traveled a lot and experienced many good times. But as more treatments and surgeries passed, he became weaker and more in pain. He lived the last year of his life completely dependent on pain medications and couldn't do much, so we were both homebound.

It's odd, but I found when we went through this trial, most of our friends stayed away. Maybe they didn't want the sadness or sorrow of "end of life." If they don't have Jesus in their life as Lord and Savior, I can see how that happens. They know what is ahead, and that is physical death. But what they don't realize is Jesus died for all of us. He is our only way to heaven! I knew and believed all this and had a peace about Jon's death because he had repented of his sins and accepted Jesus into his heart as his Lord and Savior a few days before his body died.

However, there were days I would cry out to the Lord saying I couldn't do this anymore. I was exhausted. The many pain medications turned Jon into someone I didn't even know. He was no longer the man I married but a mean and angry man addicted to pain medication. But God gave me the strength to continue. I began to mourn his death because I knew he was not going live, barring a miracle. He was very difficult to deal with and take care of. God stepped in and inspired my sister, brother, and uncle to take turns staying with me so I wasn't alone when Jon passed. I think they wanted to make sure I wasn't going to fall apart like I did when Tom passed.

What God's Word says in Philippians 4:13 is really true:

"I can do all this through him who gives me strength."

After about six long, hard years of surgeries and treatments, Jon passed. Now I had many long talks with the Lord of what was to come. I didn't want to repeat any of my mistakes or put my family through what I went through before. But this time I had time to prepare. I knew the good Lord was by my side, holding my hand the whole time. It was a huge blessing God took Jon home, with no more suffering! Now at sixty-one, I found myself widowed again.

Jon was on hospice the last few months of his life. I still took care of him, but the hospice staff helped me manage his medications and medical supplies. His nurse, Heidi, and I became good friends. She helped me understand what was happening and taught me how to care for him. Now again, I had to tell my husband it was okay to go home. My secret weapon was the grace of God as He walked me through this journey.

Then came the best part of all. I had requested a hospice chaplain for Jon, and God sent a man named Dan Olsen. He helped

Jon and I to pray and seek the Lord's will, not our will, but God's. The best news was he helped Jon receive Jesus as his Lord and Savior!! Jon passed very peacefully and went home. I was so tired but relieved Jon went home. Praise God!

For the next couple months, I was taking care of business. Now I was by myself again, feeling good at how God had worked through Dan and I to help Jon pass. But here I went again, deciding what my life was going to consist of now. I was going to be strong and NOT mess up like I did when Tom passed. My family was concerned I would go down the same path. I was good because now I had the Holy Spirit in me!!

My granddaughter Lacie came and stayed with me and did her second semester of her junior year in Chino Valley. Remember, I said I thought I had my life planned out. I was going to stay single—no marriage for me. I was going to live alone, travel, and just spend time with my family. Well again, God intervened and told me He had plans for me. He hit me upside the head and told me to trust Him.

God then put Dan Olsen back in my life. I hadn't seen him for a few months, and Heidi told me his wife had passed. Dan had told me how sick she was. I wasn't surprised she had passed. I reached out to Dan with condolences, and he invited me to her service. As it turns out, I had been searching for a church. As soon as I walked into Mountaintop Christian Fellowship, I felt I was home. I picked up the membership agreement and spent all week reading it. God kept telling me this is where He wanted me.

The following Sunday I went to church at Mountaintop. I went in the front doors, and I was welcomed and greeted in such a warm and loving way. I felt so good about being there. I did not know anyone but still felt at home. Dan saw me sitting there alone and asked if he could sit with me. He made sure he did not sit too close. After all, what would people think?

God spoke to me during praise and worship. I cried and knew I was where God wanted me. Dan asked me to lunch where we learned we had much in common, most of all, a deep love for the Lord!

When I went home, I knew by the feelings I was having that I was in trouble. I walked around the house talking to God. How could I have such feelings for Dan when I hardly knew him? If I couldn't have him, then why was I feeling like this? What was going on here? Was this God's will??

But I knew God was working in my life and would never leave me. I felt such love from my heavenly Father. I have learned through more than sixty years of trials and stumbling to trust my Lord! Not my will, but His!

What would people think of our relationship so soon after the deaths of our spouses? But these feelings I was having were undeniable. Dan and I spent a couple months getting to know each other, and it became clear God had put us together for His special purpose. We knew without a doubt we were to honor our God and get married in order to fulfill His plan for us. We obeyed, and Pastor Steve married us on March 31, 2019, at 3:31 in the afternoon.

Jeremiah 29:11–13 says:

"'For I know the plans I have for you,' declares the LORD, 'plans to prosper you and not to harm you, plans to give hope and a future. Then you will call on me and come and pray to me, and I will listen to you. You will seek me and find me when you seek me with all your heart.'"

PART 3

OUR STORY TOGETHER

CHAPTER 14

Our Greatest Gift from God

As we continue to pursue what we know to be from God, we have found what has turned out to be the greatest love in our lives. God has continually loved us and has never left us. Since we married, we have been blessed beyond measure by our awesome Lord. He has allowed us to do so many things together. We always seek to serve Him as He guides our path together. We have traveled to many places and bought and sold properties. Now He has now settled us into a beautiful home we don't deserve in Anthem Country Club. God has also blessed us with a houseboat on Lake Powell where we often enjoy the beauty of His creation. We named the houseboat "Overcomer" in honor of what the Lord has done in our lives. We are so, so blessed, and we give Him all the glory!

He has let us stumble and go through trials, but He has always been there. He has given us, in our marriage, the greatest love we have ever known. We didn't ever think our lives would be so full of love, for the Lord and for each other. In this season of our life, he has blessed us with the "love of our lives." We have an intense love for one another that we share in our "golden" years, a love we don't deserve from our heavenly Father and from one another. It's the love described in God's Word!

First Corinthians 13:4–7 says, "Love is patient, love is kind. It does not envy, it does not boast, it is not proud. It does not dishonor others, it is not self-seeking, it is not easily angered, it keeps no record of wrongs. Love does not delight in evil but rejoices with the truth. It always protects, always trusts, always hopes, always perseveres."

It doesn't stop there, though. The Lord continually blesses us through our families. We both are honored and humbled to be part of the families we married into. Our siblings and children put their love for each other above all else. We believe this is why God has blessed them all with honest and successful careers. By the grace of God, we have both been welcomed into each other's families.

In the summer of 2022, the Lord blessed us with an awesome new daughter when our son Jeff married the love of his life, Clare. We love Clare and count her as a gift from the Lord, not only for Jeff but also for us! She completes Jeff, and together they live life to the fullest, work hard, and are full of adventure. They enjoy having us be a part of their lives, and we love having them involved in ours. We have no doubt God created Jeff and Clare to live their adult lives together, married by Him, one in the flesh.

At the same time, the Lord blessed us with an awesome new grandson-to-be when Lacie, our granddaughter, became engaged to Kyle. We love Kyle and count him as a gift from God as well. His love for our granddaughter is so honorable and true. God has not only joined their hearts together but also given both Kyle and Lacie hearts to serve others through their careers as first responders. They enjoy having us be a part of their lives, and we love having them involved in ours.

The Lord has also blessed us with a bonus family, Rachel, Albert, and three beautiful boys. God put them in our lives at the perfect time. His timing is always PERFECT! We couldn't love them any more even if they were our own flesh and blood. Our lives are so full with all the kids and grandkids we have been blessed with.

The Lord has also blessed us with two different church families that have welcomed us with open arms. The Lord used Mountaintop Christian Fellowship to bring us together, and in the fall of 2022, He moved us to The Crossroads Church in Anthem, Arizona. We are currently thriving in our walk with Jesus at The Crossroads. We are coming closer to Him through small group Bible studies and serving Him as leaders in various ministries both inside and outside the church. At The Crossroads, we are His to grow and use as He sees fit.

Our journey is really one of healing through divine intervention and the power of prayer. It is a story of how God used and continues to use other people in our lives to bring us closer to Him. It is a story of accepting Jesus Christ into our hearts as our Lord and Savior, and it is a story of the Holy Spirit working within us, helping us to live as God wants us to live. Glory to God for those He places along our path!

The Holy Spirit continues to inspire us, and there is no timetable aside from His.

However, we want to be clear that we, Dan and Laurie, alone aren't doing any of this; it is God doing it through us. We give Him all the glory. It is truly an honor and a joy to be servant leaders for Him. We are humbled by all the mercy, all the grace, and all the miracles He has bestowed upon us. Yes, we are still sinners and are still tempted by the enemy. We still make mistakes. God has allowed and continues to allow trials and challenges in our lives, but we know He uses them to help us grow and get stronger for His glory. We have both persevered through long periods of tribulation where God refined us and built our character for His purposes. We are "all in" for Jesus, and that makes us better people!

James 1:2–4 says, "Consider it pure joy, my brothers and sisters, whenever you face trials of many kinds, because you know that the testing of your faith produces perseverance. Let perseverance finish its work so that you may be mature and complete, not lacking anything."

As we look back on our lives, we can say without a doubt Jesus is number one in our hearts. He has walked us down several different paths, and He has blessed us in many ways. He has never left us. He has let us stumble, but He was always there to pick us up when we asked. We always loved the Lord, though we strayed when our lives were turned upside down.

We are living proof of what God can do in our lives if we just fall to our knees and ask for forgiveness, repent, and seek the Lord for everything. We hope in some way God has, or will, use our testimony to bless others as He has us. By Christ's power, we are overcomers!

CHAPTER 15

Our Heartfelt Message to Our Readers

hank you for reading our story! It is a testament to God's love for us and of our love for those who read it. As you have read, our relationship with our Lord and Savior, Jesus Christ, is the most important part of our existence.

We believe without doubt the Bible is the infallible Word of God and is true.

We believe that both heaven and hell are real and that, as the Bible states, Jesus is the Way and the Truth and the Life. Nobody comes to the Father in heaven except through Him!

We know our bodies will die, but we will live forever in heaven because we have chosen to accept Jesus Christ as our Lord and Savior.

We have repented and turned from our sinful ways and strive to overcome the world, just as Jesus overcame the world.

We continue to prepare for our eternal destiny as we walk daily with Jesus.

We have an eternal perspective that allows us to live in peace without fear or anxiety, even though we see the world falling apart all around us.

We know by the truth of the Bible that Jesus came into this world to save us and that He is coming again to establish His new eternal kingdom. His is a kingdom that will include all those who believe in Him and accept Him into their hearts. And again, by the truth of God's Word, we know the only way to heaven is through Jesus Christ, and those who don't accept Jesus Christ will not spend eternity in heaven with their Creator, Almighty God.

We know this because Scripture is very clear in John 14:1–7 where Jesus says this:

"Do not let your hearts be troubled. You believe in God; believe also in me. My Father's house has many rooms; if that were not so, would I have told you that I am going there to prepare a place for you? And if I go and prepare a place for you, I will come back

and take you to be with me that you also may be where I am. You know the way to the place where I am going." *Thomas said to him, "Lord, we don't know where you are going, so how can we know the way?" Jesus answered, "I am the way and the truth and the life.* **No one comes to the Father except through me.** *If you really know me, you will know my Father as well. From now on, you do know him and have seen him"* (emphasis mine).

And then in John 14:25–27, Jesus states:

"All this I have spoken while still with you. But the Advocate, the Holy Spirit, whom the Father will send in my name, will teach you all things and will remind you of everything I have said to you. Peace I leave with you; my peace I give you. I do not give to you as the world gives. Do not let your hearts be troubled and do not be afraid."

The Word of God also speaks clearly to us in John 16:30–33 where Jesus's disciples were speaking to Him:

"Now we can see that you know all things and that you do not even need to have anyone ask you questions.

*This makes us believe that you came from God." "Do you now believe?" Jesus replied. "The time is coming and in fact has come when you will be scattered, each to your own home. You will leave me all alone. Yet I am not alone, for my Father is with me. I have told you these things, so that in me you may have peace. In this world you will have trouble. But take heart! **I have overcome the world***" (emphasis mine).

We love the Lord our God with all our heart, all our mind, and all our soul!

We have faith God is sovereign over all.

We believe we are nothing without Him and can do nothing apart from Him.

We believe prayer is the way to directly communicate with Jesus, and it is powerful! Every morning before we even get out of bed, we pray to Jesus.

We ask Him to empower us with the Holy Spirit so every thought, word, action, and decision we make is guided by Him. Then humbly, we trust that every thought we have, every word we say, every action we take, and every decision we make that day is guided by the Spirit of Almighty God.

Therefore, by the power of the Holy Spirit who is in us—

We choose Jesus daily!

We invite Him into our hearts daily!

We STRIVE to OVERCOME daily!

We pray you will do the same because we want to spend eternity with you.

Jesus loves you, and so do we!

— Dan & Laurie Olsen